TABLE OF CONTENTS

ACKNOWLEDGEMENTS

Grateful thanks go out to all the dedicated professionals, including but not limited to Dr Eleanor Kellon VMD, Dr Robert Bowker VMD, PhD and Gene Ovincek GPF-RMF, for generously sharing the educational resources that provide the basis for the advice in this book.

I also extend my heartfelt gratitude to all the wonderful horses that continue to teach me on my journey.

DISCLAIMER

This book does not intend to diagnose or treat without the support and advice of your vet.

Every effort has been made in the research of this book to present quality information based on the best available and most reliable sources. The author assumes no responsibility for, nor makes any warranty with respect to results that may be obtained from the procedures described. The author shall not be liable to anyone for damages resulting from reliance on any information contained within this book, whether with respect to procedures, feeding, care, treatment or remedies suggested or by reason of any mis-statement or inadvertent error contained within the pages of this book.

Readers are encouraged to always follow the guidance of professionals in their respective fields of veterinary care, farrier expertise and dietary care, seeking the relevant professional intervention as required.

FOREWORD

The aim of this book is to provide a comprehensive overview of equine laminitis in an easy to understand format. It is written for horse owners and care givers to provide them with enough knowledge to enable them to be proactive in their horse's welfare when they are suffering from laminitis.

It is only when you experience laminitis first hand that you realize just how bad it is and it is my goal to help educate so as to prevent the often devastating long-term results.

Whilst it is more work to set up a system whereby you manage your horse in a way that lowers the risk of laminitis – it is substantially less work and heartache in relation to what you would have to do to rehabilitate a laminitic animal. That old saying is definitely true: an ounce of prevention is worth a pound of cure.

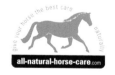

Equine Laminitis

IMMEDIATE ACTION:

What to do if your horse is currently suffering from a laminitis attack

The majority of laminitis episodes are caused by metabolic issues. If the laminitis is in both front feet, the equine is generally an easy-keeper and there is no other obvious cause such as retained placenta in a mare or a break into the feed room, then ensure that you implement the following emergency protocol as soon as possible.

- Ice the hooves or stand in a cold running stream - especially if within 8 hours of the laminitis trigger
- Remove the horse from pasture and feed only hay that has been soaked in cold water for an hour (see page 23).
  - If the horse is overweight, feed 1.5% of ideal body weight in hay per day (for a 1000 lb horse you will feed 15 lbs of hay) - NEVER go below this amount as this can lead to death from hyperlipaemia.
  - If the horse is thin, feed 2% of ideal body weight (so if horse weighs 800 lbs but should weigh 1000 lbs, feed 20 lbs of hay per day)
- Stop feeding all commercial feeds and supplements (see page 20).
- Get your vet to perform blood work for Insulin Resistance and/or Cushing's Disease and take xrays (see pages 14 and 17).
- Get your farrier to trim the hooves and use hoof boots for comfort (see pages 27-35).

Chapter One
WHAT IS LAMINITIS?

Laminitis is an extremely painful hoof condition. The actual meaning of the word "laminitis" is "inflammation of the laminae".

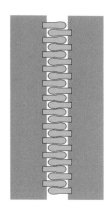

WHAT ARE LAMINAE?

In a healthy hoof the hoof wall is tightly attached to the bone inside. The bone and hoof wall both have structures call laminae attached to them and these laminae interlock with each other to form a very tight bond - imagine the bond as a closed zipper.

When your horse has laminitis there is inflammation between the two sets of laminae. This is extremely painful as unlike inflammation in soft tissue where the tissue can swell, the hoof capsule and bone are both very rigid which means that the swelling results in a huge amount of pressure that has no where to go. If you've ever hit your fingernail hard enough to bruise the tissue underneath you will have a small appreciation for the pain involved. Add to that the fact that the hooves have to support the entire weight of the horse all day long and you will see why laminitis can be so painful.

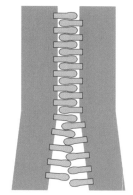

Laminitis is referred to as acute when it is in the early stages and chronic when it has been present for a long time.

FOUNDER
Many people mistakenly interchange the two words laminitis and founder but founder is more severe and occurs if the laminitis is not addressed. Founder is when the laminae detach and the connection between the bone and hoof capsule is destroyed. The hoof capsule rotates away from the bone, and in the worst cases the bone can penetrate though the bottom of the hoof.

In some horses the capsule is forced up and the bone presses down on the sole. This is known as a sinker (or distal descent) as the position of bone appears to have sunk down within the hoof capsule.

Founder is much more severe and much harder to rehabilitate than laminitis but with correct care it is fixable.

CAN IT BE PREVENTED?
YES! Despite being a common condition - according to research it ranks as the second biggest killer of horses, with colic being number one - by being vigilant you can prevent it.

Sadly there still persists a lack of education about how to treat laminitis, even amongst vets and farriers, which is why the statistics are so high. That is why horse owners need to educate themselves because they are the first line of defense against this condition.

WHICH EQUINES ARE SUSCEPTIBLE TO LAMINITIS?
Whilst ponies and some breeds such as morgans and arabs are more prone to it, unfortunately all horses, ponies and donkeys can get laminitis.

However it is preventable so being aware of the causes and being proactive in your approach to your general horse keeping will go a long way towards avoiding this painful and damaging condition.

IS MY HORSE AT RISK?
Your horse is at risk if any of the following apply:

- he's overweight
- his feet are not trimmed correctly on a regular basis
- he's turned out on lush pasture
- she's pregnant
- he's injured one leg which is forcing him to put more weight on the other three
- you feed high sugar (sweet) feed
- he's underweight but has a cresty neck
- you use shavings that may contain black walnut, as bedding
- there are black walnut trees in your horses pasture
- your horse is receiving steroid treatment
- his appetite is insatiable

PROGNOSIS
If you catch it early, before any internal damage occurs, then recovery can be expected within a month.

However, the longer it progresses, the longer the recovery. When rotation or sinking occurs you need to re-grow the hoof wall/bone connection and this can take up to nine months.

If it is chronic and internal damage is severe then there may be limitations as to how much recovery can be realistically achieved.

However, every horse is an individual and ponies especially are very hardy.

Chapter Two
ANATOMY OF THE HOOF

The horse's hoof (foot) contains a bone inside it called the coffin bone (also referred to as P3 or the pedal bone). The coffin bone is not like your typical bone. It is semi-circular in shape when looking at it from above and triangular when looking from the front or side.

COFFIN BONE (PEDAL BONE/P3)

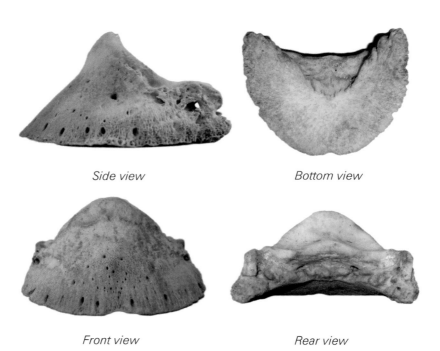

Side view

Bottom view

Front view

Rear view

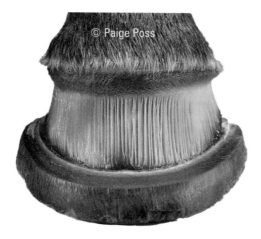

This bone forms the foundation of the hoof. Attached to the coffin bone is one set of laminae which is similar in looks to the underside of a mushroom.

Coffin bone and laminae

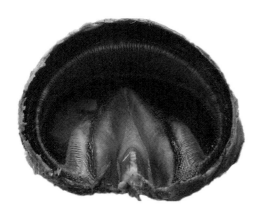

The hoof capsule, which is made up of the hoof wall, sole and frog, is the external part of the hoof that we see. It also has a set of laminae on its inside.

Hoof capsule and laminae

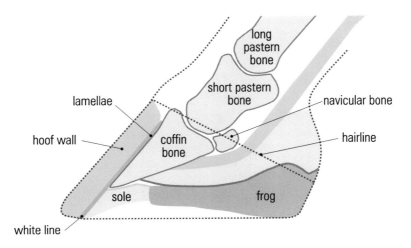

In a healthy hoof (diagram above) the coffin bone sits high in the hoof capsule (relative to the hairline) and the front edge of the coffin bone is parallel to the hoof wall at the toe. In a horse that has foundered, the bone and hoof wall are no longer parallel - see diagram below.

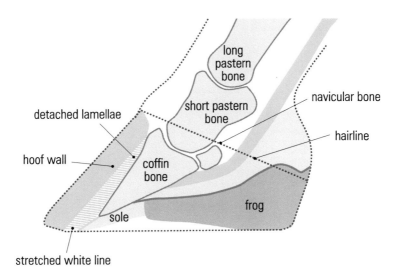

There are three bones inside the hoof capsule: the coffin bone; the short pastern; and the navicular bone.

In a healthy hoof there is a certain correlation between the external structures, such as the hairline and toe wall, and the bones.

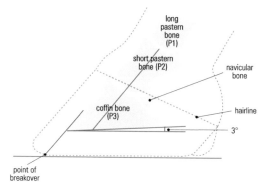

- The coffin bone is held high in the capsule, with the top-most tip being level with the hairline when viewed in on xray.

- The coffin bone and short pastern are aligned to each other so that if you were to draw a line through the center of the short pastern it would run parallel to the front edge of the coffin bone (red line).

- The front edge of the coffin bone is parallel to the hoof wall at the toe.

- The bottom edge of the coffin bone is 3-5° to the ground plane (green lines).

- The point of breakover - which is the point at which the hoof leaves the ground - is located in line with the front edge of the coffin bone (blue line).

In a hoof that has suffered from laminitis, the structures deviate from the norm.

ROTATION

When rotation occurs it can be just the capsule that rotates or it can be both the bone and the capsule that rotate.

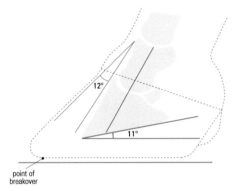

In the diagram on the right, just the capsule has rotated. We know this because the alignment of the coffin bone and short pastern has not changed. If the bone had rotated the red line would no longer be straight.

The blue lines show that the toe wall has rotated 12° away from its healthy parallel position relative to the front edge of the coffin bone. This means that the laminae have separated and the white line will be much wider than normal as a result of this.

Notice how this affects the point of breakover - it has migrated far away from its healthy location and now increases the mechanical forces on the separated hoof wall. Also the bottom edge of the coffin bone has rotated away from the ground plane.

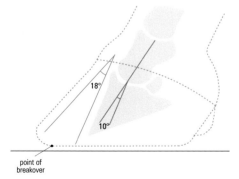

In this diagram, both the bones and the capsule have rotated.

There is 18° capsular rotation (blue lines) and 10° boney rotation (red lines). The coffin bone is also lower within the hoof capsule so this would also be classed as a sinker.

Chapter Three
SIGNS & SYMPTOMS

Laminitis most commonly occurs in the two front feet, however it can sometimes just affect one front foot or in rare cases, affect all four.

Attitude
- Depression - standing away from herd mates
- Bad behavior - such as acting lazy or not wanting to trot/canter
- Reluctance to pick up feet
- Laying down more than normal and not wanting to get up

Movement
- Reluctance to move
- Difficulty walking especially when turning
- Taking exaggerated high steps with hind legs
- Tender on gravel/rocks
- Exaggerated heel first landing
- Stiff gait

Stance
- Rocking back on heels with hind legs further under the body than normal
- Shifting weight from one foot to the other
- Tight muscles
- Anxiety and/or trembling

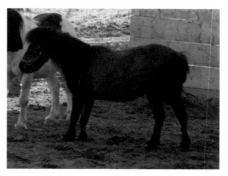

Typical founder stance - rocking back on heels to relieve pressure on the toes

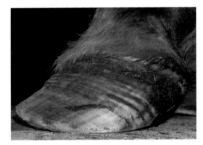

Prominent founder growth rings

Breathing
- Elevated respiration rate with pain and sweating

Pulses
- Strong, bounding pulse to the hooves

Hooves
- Excessive heat in hooves
- Bulging sole
- Pain when pressure is applied to the sole
- Prominent growth/fever rings
- Dished or flared toe wall
- Wide white line
- Blood in white line

Body condition
- Overweight or underweight but with fat pads
- Cresty neck
- Fat pads on shoulders/rump

How to take a pulse

On healthy horses it can be hard to find the pulse as it tends to be quite faint. However, all horses vary so it is wise to regularly take your own horse's pulse so that you get to know his "normal".

When there is inflammation in the hoof the pulse will feel much stronger. There will not be an increase in the speed of the pulse but it will feel a throbbing against your fingers.

If the throbbing pulse is only in one leg then it could be that the horse has an abscess or a bruise. If it is in both front legs or all four legs then suspect laminitis.

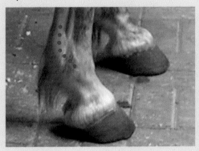

To locate the pulse, place your first two fingers just below the end of the most rearward groove that runs down the back of the leg - see red dots above.

http://www.anatomy-of-the-equine.com/equine-digital-pulses.html

SEVERITY OF LAMINITIS

Many horses have **sub-clinical laminitis** which can go unrecognized for long periods of time. The symptoms are often very mild such as a reluctance to take a canter lead, or slight tenderness on rough ground.

Sub-clinical means that it is not detectable on physical examination.

If the subclinical laminitis goes untreated it will often lead to **acute laminitis** which is when the signs and symptoms start to show up. If it is properly treated, acute laminitis can be stopped and be over in 10-14 days.

However, if not properly treated it can lead to **chronic laminitis and/or founder,** which is much harder to fix as the coffin bone and laminae can become damaged and as a result limit the chances of a full recovery.

Chronic laminitis, when not properly addressed, is often accompanied by white line disease which is where the inner hoof wall gets eaten away by fungus and bacteria. White line disease needs aggressive treatment to completely eradicate it.

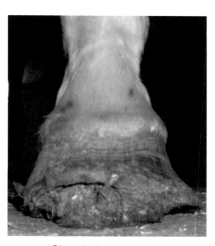

Chronic laminitis with white line disease

So it is very important to be vigilant and not let laminitis progress.

Chapter Four
LAMINITIS TRIGGERS

Accident/injury
- Injury to opposite leg

Diet
- Lush grazing/high sugar hay
- Sweet feed
- Grain overload/digestive upset

Mechanical
- LOF (Lack of Farrier)
- Poor trim

Metabolic
- Insulin resistance (Increased appetite)
- Cushing's disease (PPID)

Pregnancy
- Retained placenta

Steroid use

Stress

Systemic Infection

Chapter Five
PAIN RELIEF

ICING

In the first eight hours of a laminitis attack you may be able to prevent damage occurring if you ice the hooves or stand the horse in a cold running stream. This will help bring down the inflammation and help with the pain.

DRUGS

Phenylbutazone (Bute), Flunixin Meglumine (Banamine) and more recently, Firocoxib (Equioxx) are the three main drugs used as anti-inflammatories. Fibrocoxib has the lowest risk of gastrointestinal ulcers in short term use.

These drugs should only be used for the first 3 to 5 days of an acute laminitis attack - longer than that and they start to interfere with healing of bone and soft tissue.

If you address the cause of the laminitis and trim the hooves so that healing can take place then drugs will not be necessary to control the pain. Whilst it is hard to see an animal in agony, a certain amount of pain aids in keeping the horse relatively still so that further damage is not done.

JIAOGULAN

After the acute phase is over, the herb Jiaogulan can be very beneficial as it aids the production of nitric oxide which helps the healing process. For more information on Jiaogulan see http://www.all-natural-horse-care.com/jiaogulan-for-horses.html

Chapter Six
DIAGNOSIS

The majority of laminitis episodes are caused by metabolic issues. If the laminitis is in both front feet, the equine is generally an easy-keeper and there is no other obvious cause such as retained placenta in a mare or a break into the feed room then it is likely to be metabolic. Spring and especially fall laminitis are almost always symptomatic of metabolic issues.

Insulin Resistance (IR) is a condition where cells do not respond properly to insulin. IR horses tend to be easy keepers with a body condition score of six or higher and have fatty deposits such as a cresty neck. They are often ravenous with a large insatiable appetite.

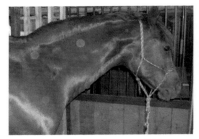

Typical cresty neck on an IR horse

The test for IR requires that a non-fasting blood sample be taken and tested for both glucose and insulin levels. The reason for non-fasting is that you need to know how your horse responds to insulin under normal conditions. Some vets will insist on you fasting your horse (based on how the test is performed in humans) so you may need to pretend that you did. However you will in fact have ensured that the horse had hay (but not grain) available at all times both the night before and the day of the test.

An additional test which is not yet widely available is leptin testing which is more sensitive than insulin and can be used to double check the insulin and glucose results. Cornell University can perform this test.

Often the blood results come back with levels that are within the lab's normal ranges. However, this does not necessarily mean that your horse doesn't have IR, as the "normal" range just means the average of all blood levels taken at that particular lab regardless of whether the specimens came from healthy animals or not.

Request a copy of the results from your vet and use the IR calculator found here http://www.freil.com/~mlf/IR/ir.html to calculate the ratio between the glucose and insulin. This will tell you if your horse is IR and how susceptible he is to laminitis.

The treatment for IR is diet and exercise - your horse will need to be kept on a strict low-sugar, balanced diet (see page 22) and once returned to soundness will benefit greatly from regular exercise.

For more information on IR visit: www.ecirhorse.org

Cushing's Disease (Pituitary Pars Intermedia Dysfunction - PPID) is a disorder of the pituitary gland that results in hormonal imbalances.

The following is a list of symptoms for Cushing's:

- Lethargy
- Muscle loss, especially across the topline
- Weight loss and pot belly appearance with patchy fat deposits on the neck and around the top of the tail
- Excessive drinking and urination
- Unexplained Fall laminitis

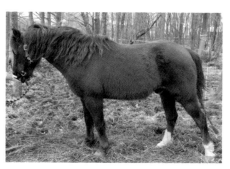

Horse with Cushing's Disease

- Either excessive sweating or failure to sweat
- Skin darkening, often with thickening and scaling
- Increased susceptibility to infections
- Poor resistance to internal parasites
- Development of allergies and hypersensitivities (e.g. vaccinations, flies)
- Infertility
- Slow spring shedding with long, coarse and sometimes curly coat with failure to shed completely occurring in advanced cases

The safest test for Cushing's is Endogenous ACTH. It requires special handling so you need to check with your vet that he is set-up to do it correctly.

Some vets will recommend you do the Dex Suppression test instead. However, this test can cause or exacerbate laminitis so is best avoided.

The treatment for Cushing's is a drug called Pergolide along with strict low-sugar, balanced diet (see page 22).

For more information on Cushing's visit: www.ecirhorse.org

Chapter Seven
RADIOGRAPHS (X-RAYS)

To properly diagnose the severity of the laminitis you need to get lateral x-rays taken. Other views are useful if damage to the bone is suspected. It is very important that these guidelines are followed:

MARKERS
Many vets do not routinely use markers when x-raying the hooves but without them it is hard to be accurate with the diagnosis and subsequent trim. You can apply them yourself prior to the x-rays being taken.

Toe wall - this marker is crucial in measuring rotation and location of the coffin bone. Attach a flexible piece of wire or chain from the junction of the toe wall and hairline down the center of the toe wall to the point of breakover. Light pull chain works well. Use duct tape to securely attach to the hoof wall.

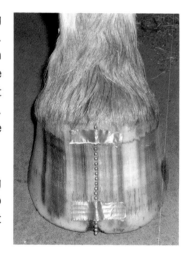

Frog tip - this marker is vital in calculating where to trim the breakover.Use a thumb tack to mark the tip of the frog (the furthest point away from the heels on the frog).

WEIGHT BEARING
If possible the hooves need to be weight bearing - ideally with the opposite hoof held up.

TRUE LATERALS
The x-ray machine should be parallel to the hoof and the beam aimed at the center of the coffin bone so as to avoid distortion.

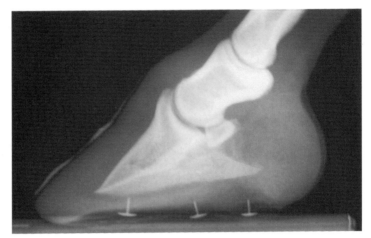

Example of a good x-ray above - the toe marker accurately follows the hoof wall and the frog has been clearly marked with three thumb tacks. Also it is a true lateral as the two wings of the coffin bone line up (yellow shaded area).

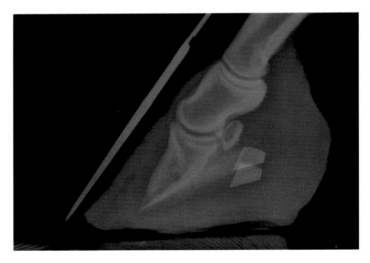

Example of a not so good x-ray above - the toe marker is not suitable as it is rigid and not following the contours of the hoof wall and goes well above the hairline. There is no marker on the frog and it is not a true lateral as both wings of the coffin bone can be seen.

READING X-RAYS

The first x-ray shows a relatively healthy hoof. The alignment between the bones is good and although there is no hoof wall marker, the coffin bone appears to be parallel to the hoof wall.

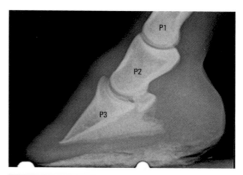

The second x-ray is of a very deformed coffin bone. It is from a chronically laminitic pony and over half of the coffin bone is missing from the bottom edge. There is also a large amount of remodelling at the front of the coffin bone. This is as a result of having a high heeled trim and uncontrolled laminitis for many years.

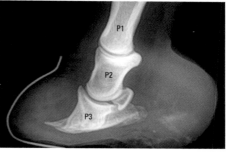

Below are photos taken of the same hoof prior to the x-ray. In the one on the right I have overlaid the x-ray to show the position of the bones within the hoof. As you can see the coffin bone has sunk down so far that the entire short pastern bone is within the hoof capsule. With this much damage to the bone the hoof will never look normal, however this pony is still thriving with careful management and the use of hoof boots (see photos on page 26).

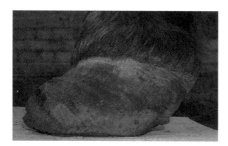
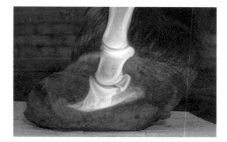

Chapter Eight
DIET

Laminitis is becoming a very common condition these days, mostly due to the lush pastures that more and more horses and ponies are being grazed on.

Horses are classed as foragers/grazers which means that their digestive systems are designed to cope with a continuous supply of small amounts of roughage at a time - their relatively small stomach and large gut are perfectly suited for this. In their natural habitat, they often have to travel great distances to obtain food and water and the wild grasses that they feed on are low in nutrition so they graze for at least 18-20 hours per day.

In comparison domestic horses have access to large amounts of high nutrient grasses and are confined to much smaller areas. This results in a horse who consumes more carbohydrates (sugars) than its body can handle - as it's not burning them off with movement - and this is often the biggest contributing factor in causing laminitis.

Also many stable-kept horses are given large amounts of grain in one feeding and then left for long periods of time with nothing in their stomach. This is very disruptive to the digestive system and can contribute to laminitis.

Grain is not easily digested by the horse as it did not encounter it in the wild so the digestive system is not evolved to cope with it. Also many commercial feeds and supplements have high amounts of sugars in them, making them unsuitable for the laminitic horse.

The most appropriate diet to feed to a horse is grass or grass hay on a free choice basis. However, due to current farming practices which aim to increase the nutritional value of pasture grasses, many fields are now too rich in sugars for safe grazing. This means that you may have to restrict the amount of grass available to your horse.

GRAZING MUZZLE

For some horses, using a grazing muzzle can be a good solution to this problem. The muzzle is designed to reduce the amount of grass that the horse can eat whilst still allowing it to be with its herd mates.

PADDOCK PARADISE

Another option is to set up a Paddock Paradise track system. This allows you to creatively engage your horse in more movement whilst restricting grazing at the same time.

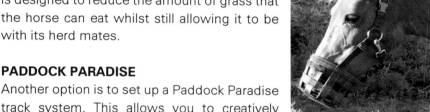

Grazing muzzle

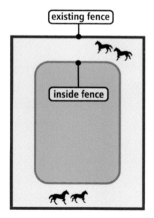

Paddock Paradise is based on wild horse studies and its basic concept is to make a track for your horse instead of just providing a big open space.

By installing an additional inside fence to your current fencing situation a track can be created. The track encourages more movement and gives you the opportunity to make a more stimulating environment than a regular dry lot. Visit http://www.all-natural-horse-care.com/paddock-paradise.html for more information.

HAY

If your horse is sensitive, it may need to be kept off pasture completely. Grass hay is a much safer alternative to pasture and when fed in a slow feeder it is possible to ensure that it available to your horse throughout the day and night (for more information on slow feeders visit http://www.all-natural-horse-care.com/horse-slow-feeder.html).

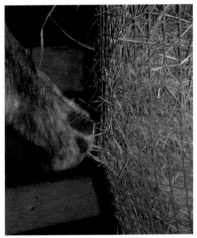

However, not all hay is low in sugar so it is best get your hay tested to see if it is suitable.

Slow feeder hay net

HAY TESTING

If your horse's laminitis if due to metabolic issues it is important to get your hay tested to make sure that the combined total of both sugar and starch is below 10%. Some hay suppliers test their hay, so it is always worth asking your supplier if they know the percentage of sugar in their hay.

If not, you need to get hold of a corer to take the sample - many feed stores and some agricultural extension offices have them and will loan them out. For best results take samples from at least 15-20 bales.

Send the sample off for analysis - specifying wet chemistry as it is more accurate than NIR - and choose a package that also tests for both major and trace minerals (specifically calcium, magnesium, phosphorus, copper, zinc and manganese). That way you can custom mineral balance your hay to ensure your horse is getting everything it needs. Equi-analytical's 603 trainer package is a good one and costs around $49 (www.equi-analytical.com).

In the meantime it is safest to soak your hay in clean, warm water for 30 minutes (or for an hour in cold water) before feeding as this will reduce the sugar levels by up to 30%.

Once you have the results you can check to see what the sugar levels are. For horses, the sugars that affect them the most are the ESCs (Ethanol Soluble Carbohydrates). Many people still think that it's the WSCs (Water Soluble Carbohydrates) that are of concern but they are just the amount of sugars available to the plant itself.

When digested, starch is converted to sugar so by adding the percentage of ESC to the percentage of starch we get the total sugar in the hay. For most metabolic horses the combined total needs to be below 10%, but for some it needs to be below 8%.

SUPPLEMENTS

Finding an "off the shelf" supplement that provides the missing nutrients for your hay can be tricky. Many supplements don't contain the correct ratio of minerals to balance your hay, and if the ratio between minerals is incorrect the body won't be able to use them properly and this could lead to other problems.

The most cost-effective solution is to design a custom mineral supplement. Companies like HorseTech (http://www.horsetech.com/) or Uckele (http://equine.uckele.com/) will do this for you.

Alternatively you can learn how to do it yourself by taking an online course with Dr Kellon (http://www.drkellon.com/). There is a steep learning curve to ensure that you do it properly but in the long run you will save money. If you do decide to do it yourself please make sure you fully understand the calculations, and order the correct amounts of each mineral, as some of the minerals are toxic in excessive dosages and could cause serious harm.

Chapter Nine
WEIGHT MANAGEMENT

We are all so used to seeing fat horses these days that we have come to accept "fat" as "normal". Additional weight puts your horse at a higher risk for laminitis.

To maintain weight a horse or pony should get approx 2% of its body weight in hay per day. To lose weight you can reduce this to 1.5%.

Never go any lower than 1.5% as you could cause hyperlipaemia, which is a condition where there are abnormally high levels of fat or lipids in the blood. It is often fatal.

Using the Henneke Body Condition Scoring method, an ideal weight is a score of 5-6 where you should be able to easily feel the ribs.

Fatty deposits on the neck, withers and rump can be signs of a metabolic issue.

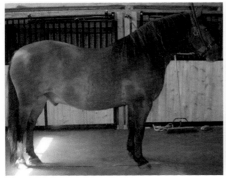

Obese horse
body condition score 9+

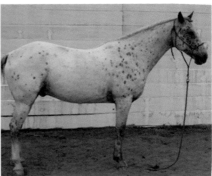

Healthy horse
body condition score 6

HENNEKE SCALE - BODY CONDITION SCORES

Score	Description
1. Poor	Extremely emaciated; no fatty tissue; vertebrae, ribs, tail head, and bones of withers, shoulder, and neck are visible
2. Very Thin	Emaciated; slight tissue cover over bones; vertebrae, ribs, tail head, and bones of withers, shoulder, and neck are visible
3. Thin	Slight fat cover over body; individual vertebrae and ribs no longer visibly discernible; withers, shoulders, and neck do not appear overly thin
4. Moderately Thin	Ridge of spine and outline of ribs are visible; tail head may or may not be visible depending on the breed; withers, shoulders, and neck do not appear overly thin
5. Moderate	Spine and ribs cannot be seen, however ribs can be felt; tail head is spongy; withers, shoulders, and neck are rounded and smooth
6. Moderately Fleshy	Slight crease down spine; ribs and tail head feel spongy; fat deposits along withers and neck and behind shoulders
7. Fleshy	Crease down spine; ribs have fat filling between them; tail head spongy; fat deposits along withers and neck and behind shoulders
8. Fat	Apparent crease down spine; ribs difficult to feel; soft fat surrounding tail head; fat deposits along withers, behind shoulders, and on inner thighs; neck is large
9. Extremely Fat	Obvious crease down spine; patchy fat on ribs; bulging fat on tail head, withers, behind shoulders, and on neck; fat fills in flank and on inner thighs

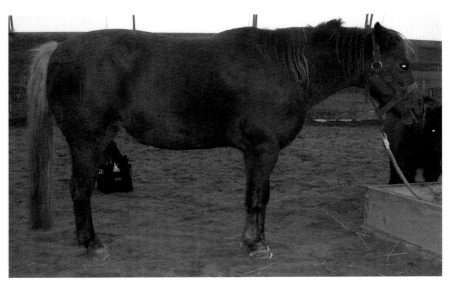

Obese pony (BCS 9) above - note the square rump, rotund belly and overall extra padding. Same pony below at her ideal weight (BCS 6).

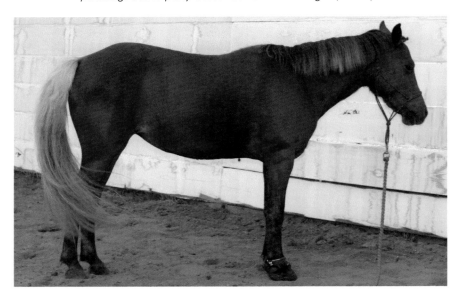

Chapter Ten
HOOF CARE

If your horse has its feet trimmed properly on a regular basis, it has a much better chance of withstanding a laminitis attack. Lack of proper hoof care is one of the leading contributors to laminitis.

A good trim allows the hoof capsule to form the strongest bond possible with the coffin bone via the laminae. Excessive heel or toe length will prevent this from happening.

A good trim also encourages, through correct stimulation, healthy horn quality, robust frogs and well developed internal structures which enable the hoof to function properly.

Shoes are often detrimental to a healthy hoof as they don't allow it to function as nature intended, but if you feel you have to put shoes on your horse then ensuring the trim is correct is a step in the right direction. However, I would highly recommend against using shoes on a horse suffering from laminitis. Not only is it painful to have nails hammered into an already inflamed hoof but it also limits the adjustments you can make to return the hoof to health. When the connection between the coffin bone and the hoof wall fails the best thing to do is to relieve the pressure on the walls. It is impossible to do this with shoes.

WHEN TO TRIM?
If the hoof form is perfect at the time of a laminitis attack then a trim may not be immediately necessary. But it is vitally important to keep the hoof in optimal shape during the whole episode and thereafter.

If the hoof is not in perfect shape, then the sooner you can get the trim done the better. Even if this means trimming the hooves whilst the horse is lying down.

A physiologically correct trim will ensure that the hoof mechanics work with the hoof, not against it. It will enable the hoof to start healing and encourage a tight connection between the coffin bone and hoof wall as it regrows.

If you cannot get a competent trimmer out to your horse straightaway, then be sure to cushion the hooves with either temporary pads (see page 33) or hoof boots with pads in. This will alleviate some of the mechanical strain on the lamina by transferring some of the horse's weight to the sole and frog.

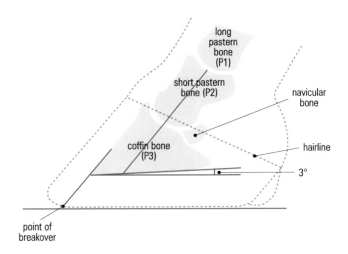

DE-ROTATING TRIM

If your horse has rotation, then a de-rotating trim is needed to restore the hoof to a form that will promote recovery.

When the capsule and/or bone rotate out of their healthy position your farrier will have to adjust the way he trims to compensate for it. This is where xrays become important.

The aim of the de-rotating trim is to return the coffin bone and hoof capsule to a healthy state, where:

- The coffin bone is held high in the capsule, with the top-most tip being level with the hairline when viewed on xray.

- The coffin bone and short pastern are aligned to each other so that if you were to draw a line through the center of the short pastern it would run parallel to the front edge of the coffin bone (red line).

- The front edge of the coffin bone is parallel to the hoof wall at the toe.

- The bottom edge of the coffin bone is 3-5° to the ground plane (green lines).

- The point of breakover - which is the point at which the hoof leaves the ground - is located in line with the front edge of the coffin bone (blue line).

Below is an example using an xray and photo of the same hoof to show the existing hoof compared to how it will look after the first de-rotating trim.

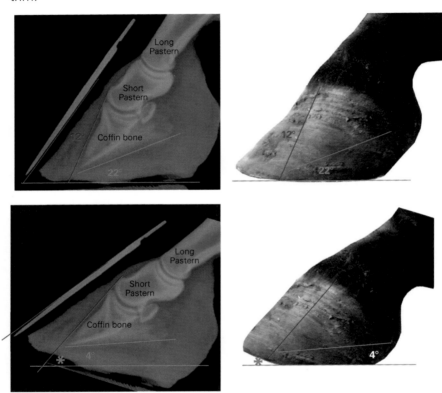

On this hoof, the heel is very high so by lowering the heel using an 18° angle (22° minus 4°) this de-rotates the bottom edge of the coffin bone back to 4° relative to the ground.

When doing the de-rotating trim, care must be taken to ensure that the toe area of the hoof is not touched at all from the bottom (sole side - see blue asterisk) as the sole underneath the tip of the coffin bone is often too thin.

READING THE HOOF

Trimming to xrays is by far the best way to correct hoof pathology. However, if xrays are not available there are certain clues that can be used to aid with trimming.

When studying photos of hooves the top 1/2" of growth (just below the hairline) will almost always be healthy, even in a rotated hoof. The angle of this growth can be used to project where the hoof wall should be.

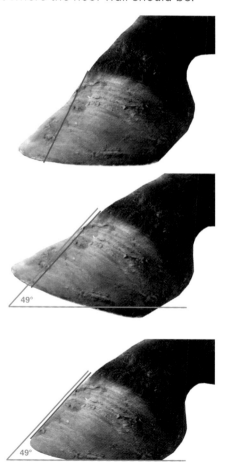

So if we draw a line (red line on top photo) parallel to this growth we can estimate where the healthy toe wall would be.

Studies have shown that in most front hooves, the angle between the front edge of the coffin bone and the ground is 45°. In wild horse studies the bottom edge of the coffin bone is generally 3-5° to the ground. So if we take 4° as average, a healthy toe wall will be approx 49° to the ground (45° plus 4° equals 49°).

By rotating the photo so that the red and green lines become parallel we can get a good indication of the angle that the heel needs to be trimmed.

When using this method, extreme caution should be taken and the trim should only be performed by an experienced professional.

Chapter Eleven
HOOF BOOTS

Hoof boots are often necessary for a horse with laminitis as they provide comfort and protection until the hoof has healed. There are many different boots available but some of the most popular for rehab are the Softride Comfort Boot, the Easyboot RX, the Jogging Shoes and the Easyboot Epic.

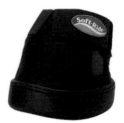
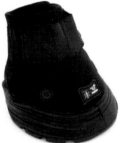

Softride Comfort Boots　　*Easyboot RX*

The Softrides and RXs are both purely rehab boots and are very good for extremely foundered hooves, whereas the Jogging Shoes and Epics can be used for riding as well. Visit www.all-natural-horse-care.com/hoof-boots.html for more information on all the boots currently available.

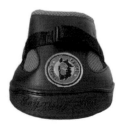
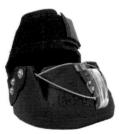

Equine Jogging Shoes　　*Easyboot Epic*

EMERGENCY HOOF BOOTS

If you are unable to get hoof boots for your horse you can make a temporary boot very easily using duct tape and foam pads. The foam does squash down after a couple of days (although some foam can be revived by placing near a heat source for a while) so you will need to replace it quite frequently but it's great to get you through an emergency.

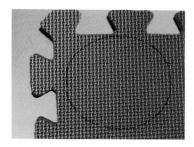

Using a foam puzzle piece (these are sold as a mat for home gyms or children's play areas at stores such as Walmart), place the horse's hoof on the foam and trace around it to get the correct size and shape.

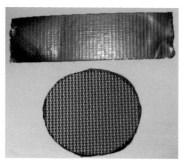

Cut out the foam and then cut three pieces of duct tape that are approx 4" longer than the foam cut out. If it is for a small pony then cut it 3".

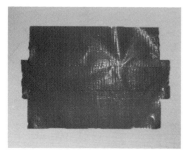

Layer the three strips of duct tape so that they overlap each other by approx 3/4" - one in the center and one either side.

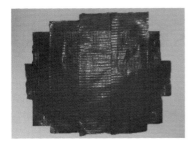

Cut another three strips of duct tape, turn them 90° and layer them over the first three.

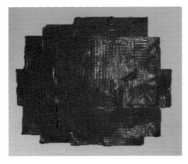

Cut another three strips of duct tape, turn them 90° and layer them over the second layer.

If the horse is still mobile you may want to add a couple more layers to make them more durable.

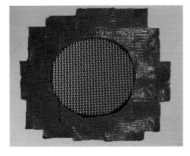

Place your foam cut out in the center of the duct tape.

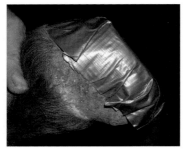

Lift the horse's hoof and make sure it is clean and dry. Keeping the foot raised, place the foam pad on the sole of the hoof and quickly stick down the duct tape around the hoof wall.

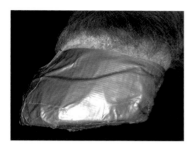

Then place the hoof on the ground and wrap two more strips of duct tape around the whole hoof to secure the edges. Make sure you keep it below the hairline.

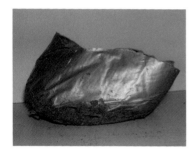

To remove the boot, make two vertical tears in the duct tape, one either side of the heels. This will allow you to slip the boot off without ruining it. The boot can then be reapplied and secured with another couple of strips of duct tape.

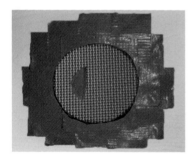

As an alternative, if your horse is particularly sore in the area under the tip of the coffin bone, you can cut away some of the pad to relieve the pressure in that area.

Chapter Twelve
EXERCISE

It is very important for horses to move, so avoid confining your laminitic horse to a stall. Give him an area that is big enough for him to move around in if he wants too (ideally at least 60 x 60 ft). Provide a nice deep bed in one corner so that he is comfortable when he lies down but keep the footing in the rest of the area relatively firm. This will encourage better hoof mechanism and aid in healing.

Pea gravel (approx 1/2") is a great option for horses. It makes a very comfortable bed (think of it as a big bean bag and the way you can wiggle around to make it mold so you are perfectly supported) and provides relief for sore hooves. It needs to be at least 4-6 inches deep so that it can deform under the horse's weight and not cause pressure points.

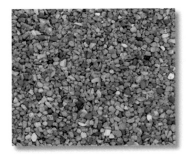

If the laminitis is very bad, your horse will probably not want to move much in the initial stages but it is important to give him the option. As he starts to feel better his movement will increase.

Never force a horse to move if he is too uncomfortable, but hand walking for 5-10 minutes twice a day is very beneficial when he is more comfortable.

Once your horse is sound it is important to ensure that he gets regular exercise. Ideally work him up to 30 minutes of trotting per day or at least every other day. Be sure to warm up and down with 5 minutes of walking.

Chapter Thirteen
FURTHER INFORMATION

If you wish to learn more there are many online resources available. Below are some recommendations.

Information on keeping horses healthy through natural horse care
http://www.all-natural-horse-care.com

Educational material featuring high quality dissection photos
http://www.anatomy-of-the-equine.com

Learn how to read the hoof
http://www.ironfreehoof.com

Detailed information on Equine Cushing's Disease and Insulin Resistance
http://ecirhorse.org

Laminitis articles on Gene Ovnicek's website
http://www.hopeforsoundness.com/cms/categories/information/lameness.html

Information on slow feeding and paddock paradise tracks
http://paddockparadise.wetpaint.com

Information on safer grazing practices
http://www.safergrass.org

Information on treating laminitis without the use of horseshoes
http://www.naturalhorsetrim.com

General information on laminitis
http://www.thelaminitissite.org

CPSIA information can be obtained
at www.ICGtesting.com
Printed in the USA
LVIC04n1431231115
463836LV00021B/233